PRAISE FOR

POP

50 Amazing Secrets to a Successful Labor & Delivery or C-section

"A new mother herself and a law professor, Peery has gathered advice from more than 80 new mothers in this slim volume to create an alternative to the textbook-like pregnancy titles. The 50 tips in this work touch on everything from packing for the hospital to recovering from labor and discuss various options, including water birth, medicated births, and C-sections. Each tip includes two or three stories from real moms that show the wide range of normal when it comes to childbirth and offer advice that readers might not get elsewhere."

—Library Journal

"It provides advice on everything from what to take to the hospital during labor to the pros and cons of epidurals. However, this book stands out due to its encouraging, nonjudgmental tone. Peery says up front that she's no expert, but this fact makes her book all the more appealing. Readers will feel from the get-go that she's on their side, rooting for them. Mostly, she quotes other women, who offer stories and advice about their own birth experiences. Pregnant readers who finish this book will likely feel more knowledgeable and more secure about what's ahead. A solid, supportive advice book to help women through the physical and mental work of childbirth."

—Kirkus Reviews

"A woman can read a dozen pregnancy books before giving birth and still find herself lost once the process actually begins. What do contractions really feel like? How long do different stages of labor last? Do epidurals really work? How does one handle the pain without one? Pamela Peery didn't realize how ill-prepared she was for giving birth until labor was upon her, and the experience inspired her to collect the advice and stories of others. The result is POP: 50 Amazing Secrets to a Successful Labor & Delivery or C-Section. This slim volume is packed with quotes from more than eighty women regarding their own experiences with having a baby. No matter what questions you might have, whether you're expecting your first or have already been through birth before, this book is sure to provide some inspiration. What should you bring to the hospital? Find ideas that might not be included on other lists. Curious about early labor? Get some ideas about what to expect. Read the thoughts of women who have had epidurals—they usually work, and you can still push even when you're numb—as well as of women who have gone all natural—remember that your body is made to give birth. POP would make a great gift to any expectant mama."

—**San Francisco Book Review**

"The perfect 'must have' for every expectant mom. Reading these honest and short tips from moms all over the world is a fantastic and easy way for women to prepare for childbirth."

—**Christine Goldman, CD, CPD, CBE, LE.** *Certified birth doula, childbirth educator and owner of Doulas of Central New York*

"How come no one wrote this before? It seems so obvious, but there's nothing else out there like this book."

—**Joanne B.,** *Bryn Mawr, PA*

"A tremendous book. Great for dads. Funny too."

—**Gregory K.,** *Philadelphia, PA*

"Great book. Wonderful and helpful tips from the real experts—real moms! A must-have for all expectant moms and dads. I can't wait to be able to give my daughter this book when her time comes."

—**Joy C.,** *Hingham, MA*

POP

50 AMAZING SECRETS

to a SUCCESSFUL LABOR & DELIVERY or C-SECTION

BY PAMELA PEERY

CASSIDY PRESS

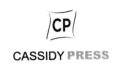

CASSIDY PRESS

POP

50 AMAZING SECRETS
TO A SUCCESSFUL LABOR & DELIVERY OR C-SECTION

First published by Cassidy Press in the United States, May 2014

NOTE: This book is intended only as a general guide for those
seeking to know more about health issues relating to childbirth,
labor and delivery. It is not intended to substitute for, conflict with,
or countermand the advice of your qualified health care provider.
The author and publisher accept no responsibility for readers' use
of the information contained herein.

Cataloguing in Publication Data
Peery, Pamela
POP: 50 Amazing Secrets to a Successful Labor & Delivery
or C-section / by Pamela Peery

p.   cm.

ISBN 978-0-9886801-0-4

1. Childbirth 2. Labor and delivery 3. Vaginal delivery and C-section
4. Comments—of new mothers for new mothers I. Title: 50 Amazing Secrets
to a Successful Labor & Delivery or C-section II. Title.

RG525.L873   2013
618.4'5–dc23   2012923368

For orders or information contact:

CASSIDY PRESS

806 E. AVENIDA PICO, STE I-163
SAN CLEMENTE, CA 92673

cassidypressbooks.com | info@cassidypressbooks.com

Cover design by Lynne Door & Bridget Hostert
Interior design by Susanne Weibl & Bridget Hostert

"**W**omen suffered through the agonies and dangers of birthing together, sought each other's support and shared the relief of successful deliveries.... This 'social childbirth' experience united women."

—Leavitt, Judith Walzer.
Brought to Bed: Childbearing in America, 1750 to 1950.
Oxford University Press, 1988

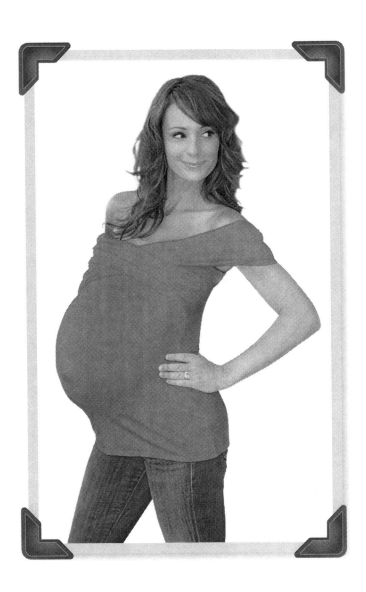

Dedicated

to the expectant mother

who might feel

a little rattled

by the prospect of giving birth

* * * * *

This book represents moms all over the world

holding your hand

& cheering you on

Welcome to motherhood

READ THIS FIRST

The stories and tips in this book are not intended or implied to be medical advice nor any kind of substitute for professional medical opinions.

This book is also not intended to be a complete list of possible scenarios or solutions.

Childbirth is a serious life or death event **unique** to every woman and requires hands-on and careful monitoring from medical professionals who are qualified to assess your unique situation. The information provided is for educational purposes and its accuracy is not guaranteed. You understand and agree that neither Pamela Peery, Cassidy Press, nor anyone associated with this book are responsible or liable for any claim, loss or damage of any kind directly or indirectly resulting from any use of this information.

These quotes are edited quotes from real women, extracted by me from the birth story each sent me. All names have been changed. The outcomes they experienced applied to their unique situations and bodies. **Do not attempt** anything described in this book without your doctor's permission and supervision. You **must consult** your medical doctor or other qualified medical professional regarding every phase and event of your pregnancy, labor and vaginal delivery or C-section.

Thank you.

IN
THIS
BOOK

THIS IS IT—THE MOMENT you've been waiting for your whole life. You've endured and, hopefully, enjoyed many months of pregnancy and are ready to give birth. You are finally going to have your precious baby.

What happens now?

All women know the classic movie and TV scenarios: you are out walking somewhere and your water breaks. (Just a little, of course—no big messes for TV or movie girl.) You calmly put your hand on your husband's arm, say "Honey, it's time," and catch a cab to the hospital.

Or you're lying in bed and feel slightly unpleasant twinges. You turn to your husband and announce, "I think this is it." Then you gracefully gather your neatly packed bags and your husband drives you to the hospital, while you sit dreaming of your new baby.

Both scenarios end a short time later with you pushing on a nice crisp hospital bed, where you turn a little red and puff a few times until you hear your baby cry. The doctor triumphantly lifts the infant up, announces the gender, and *voilà*—that's it! Easy peazy.

Is that how it's going to happen, you wonder excitedly?

No, not exactly.

I started this book after my own birthing experience. The labor chapters of my pregnancy books and my hospital's childbirth-preparation class did little to equip me for labor. I thought I was ready. After all—I took a labor and delivery class, asked my ob/gyn a gazillion questions and read the labor portion of the pregnancy books I'd had lying around.

I'm prepared! Let's go—I'm ready to roll.

Fast forward to a shot of me after 30 hours of painful "early labor"—excruciating, steady contractions that were only supposed to last a handful of hours. Frantic readings and re-readings of the early labor pages of my pregnancy guides and hospital's childbirth preparation handbook ("doesn't it say *anywhere* that this could last *so long*?") after being sent home from the hospital for "false" labor twice (yes—two times) made me wonder if I was the only woman ever to have gone through this.

Where was *my* experience in these books? Why was I left in the dark? Why didn't anyone *tell* me this could happen in normal labor?

How could the Internet age—where news travels at the speed of light and every celebrity kiss from Hollywood to Bali flashes onto our computer screens instantly—leave me in the dark about childbirth? Trillions of women before me have had babies. Where is this repository of knowledge? Where is *their* wisdom?

If I hadn't been so swept up by the wonderful creature clutching at my bosom, I would have devoted that first year to getting my money back for the class and giving the pregnancy book authors a *piece of my mind*.

Lucky for them I was busy.

I did, however, create a website requesting women's labor stories. I got the word out that I was writing a book about what labor is like in the real world—what women wished they'd known beforehand, what they will do differently next time.

The ultimate childbirth expert? A new mom.

I spent the next few years pulling myself out of bed at 3 a.m. a few mornings a week and sneaking downstairs to my computer to pour over labor and C-section stories from women around the world—in the dark, while my family slept. With tears in my eyes and darkness all around, I got to relive the most wondrous and intimate moments of women I'd never met or even spoken to.

Turns out I wasn't the only one who didn't experience "textbook" labor. I began to wonder if there was any such thing as a "typical" childbirth.

In the end, although we were strangers, I felt like these new moms and I were friends united with a common goal: to share our stories and wisdom with *you*, so you would be better prepared than we were.

This book represents more than 80 women reaching across time and space to hold your hand. Soothe and reassure you. Laugh with you. Encourage and advise you. And hopefully make your labor or C-section a better experience than ours was.

Enjoy.

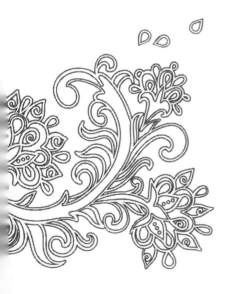

1 ADVICE AND ENCOURAGEMENT—
CHOOSING WHAT TO PACK

Packing for a hospital stay is not familiar territory for most women. After procrastinating until the last possible second, I forced myself to pack a few things—change of clothing for me, some books, a sweet outfit for my newborn and some snacks. Yet later at the hospital, I found myself wishing I'd brought other things.

Here are some items moms were happy they'd packed or wished they'd brought to the hospital:

- magazines
- camera
- small mirror
- baggy or stretchy pants
- nice clothes *(one set for hospital photograph)*
- cute baby blanket & hat
- favorite soap
- maternity nightgown

- fuzzy socks
- breast pads
- nursing bra *(if you're breastfeeding)*
- lip balm

TIP #1

. . . .

BRING MAGAZINES, A CAMERA AND
A SMALL MIRROR TO THE HOSPITAL

Someone suggested that I bring magazines to the hospital, and I'm so happy I did. Although I also brought a book, I kept picking up a magazine instead. I just couldn't concentrate enough to read my book. Plus I didn't have to try to remember where I left off or what had previously happened.

—Andrea

The things that I would have done differently with this labor is—I should have brought a camera. I forgot to pack my camera and didn't realize it until my husband was cutting the umbilical cord.

—LeeAnn

I wish I had a mirror to see my son being born. I didn't think I wanted one, but thinking back it would have been nice to see.

—Stacey

When the head crowned, the midwives got a mirror so I could see the head. That helped me a lot in pushing out my baby.

—Lisa

TIP #2

....

DON'T FORGET NICE CLOTHES FOR EVERYONE YOUR FAVORITE SOAP AND BAGGY PANTS

I'm so glad I brought some cute baby hats and baby blankets to the hospital, including one that matched her "picture" outfit. The swaddling blankets at the hospital are functional, but not pretty, and they'll be wrapped in that blanket and wearing the hospital's hat in your hospital picture unless you bring your own.

—Penny

After delivery, taking a shower with citrus scented bath gel made me feel incredibly human.

—Gabriella

Don't bring the pant size you wore before getting pregnant—chances are you won't be going home in them.

—Ayn

TIP #3

. . . .

PACK A MATERNITY NIGHTGOWN
AND YOUR FAVORITE SOCKS

Pajamas with pants are a poor choice. Get a nightgown (maternity!) so nurses can easily assist you and you can more easily take care of post-partum needs.

—Gabriella

I'm so glad I brought my favorite fuzzy socks with me to the hospital. They kept my feet warm and cozy during labor, and I didn't feel so naked even though I was only wearing a thin hospital gown. They were like a security blanket for my feet.

—Penny

TIP #4

. . . .

YOU'LL ALSO NEED BREAST PADS
LIP BALM AND YOUR NURSING BRA
(if you're breastfeeding)

I wish I was told to bring breast pads to the hospital. I am sure they had them, but it would have been a whole lot easier to have them myself than to have to wait for someone to bring them to me. I leaked everywhere.

—Lucille

My lips were getting so chapped and the skin was peeling off them. Friends told me to make sure to take ChapStick with me, but I forgot.

—Theresa

I'm glad my sister told me to bring some lip balm with me to the hospital. I remember asking Russell to put it on my lips about every 20 minutes while I was in labor. My lips were getting so dry. I'm also happy I remembered my nursing bra.

—Andrea

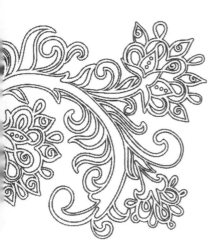

2 ADVICE AND ENCOURAGEMENT—
JUMP-STARTING LABOR NATURALLY
IF YOU'RE PAST DUE

Ok, so you've been pregnant a long time. Are you past 40 weeks and ready to have that baby now? Were you ready last year, it seems? Yes, girlfriend, first pregnancies often go past 40 weeks. Sorry.

But there could be a glimmer of hope. Thankfully, some women have seemingly jump-started their labor by:

- stimulating their nipples *(with close monitoring by qualified medical professional and doctor's approval)*

- having sex

- using a breast pump *(with close monitoring by qualified medical professional and doctor's approval)*

- walking

TIP #5
....

STIMULATING NIPPLES CAN BRING ON LABOR
(with doctor's approval)

Just two days into my much anticipated vacation, I went into labor. Actually, my water started leaking on Monday, but it was just dribbles. So we waited until morning to make sure it was my water. It sped up on Tuesday morning, so we started self-inducing methods. I started doing nipple stimulation—1 minute on, 4 minutes resting. That is what put me into immediate regular contractions. They went from 7 minutes apart to 2 minutes apart.

—Lori

TIP #6

··········

INTERCOURSE OR WALKING
CAN STIMULATE CONTRACTIONS

If I could do things differently, I would try more things at home to induce labor naturally. I walked and exercised like crazy, but to no avail. I will try intercourse with my next pregnancy if the baby is overdue. I know many people, coincidentally or otherwise, who had luck with this method.

—Traci

We knew that walking could help a labor to progress so we seized the opportunity to get some fresh air. Apparently walking works VERY well. The leash had barely been slipped off of Max's neck when my contractions were renewed at a substantial pace.

—Katya

My 38 week doctor's appointment was on a Tuesday, and the doctor said I was not dilated at all and that he'd see me in a week. Although I was disappointed not to have made any progress I figured at least my husband and I would have one more weekend to relax and be alone. So that Thursday evening we went out to a friend's softball game. We got home around 11 p.m. and decided that it'd be a good idea to have sex, maybe for the last time for a while. Afterwards we fell asleep. But at 2 a.m. I woke up to pain in my abdomen, like horrible menstrual cramps. I immediately knew what was happening ... I was in labor.

—Stacey

TIP #7

. . . .

SOME WOMEN USE BREAST PUMPS
TO INDUCE LABOR
(with doctor's approval)

Once I was done eating Tina suggested I start using the breast pump since my contractions were not seeming as intense. So we got it out and hooked it up, and let's just say it worked. I would literally have it on for a few seconds and a contraction would come on. After about 2 or 3 of these I decided that my labor was progressing just fine without the added help, and had them put it away.

—Heather

3 ADVICE AND ENCOURAGEMENT—
THE INITIAL STAGE OF LABOR

Some of the most fundamental things first-time pregnant women want to know are: How will I know I'm in "real" labor? When I go into labor, what will it feel like? Will the contractions start slowly, or come on quickly?

Like most first-time moms, I expected the onset of labor to be obvious. Contractions would be instantly recognizable—like you see in the movies, right? Maybe. The initial stage of labor (sometimes called "early labor") can be subtle, come in spurts, last for days and surprise you in other ways.

Labor and contractions are experienced differently by every woman— and the variations are numerous. Ask your doctor for a list of labor symptoms and call him or her immediately if they begin to occur.

Here are some experiences of other women:

- contractions may feel like sharp pains, cramps, or a tightening
- they might be felt in your back, legs, hips or buttocks
- they may stop and start
- the hospital might send you home
- early labor could last for days

TIP #8

. . . .

REALIZE THAT CONTRACTIONS
FEEL DIFFERENT TO DIFFERENT PEOPLE

I have to say contractions were MUCH different than I'd imagined—a bit like Braxton Hicks and menstrual cramps mixed.

—Althea

For me, my entire abdomen got really tight and hard to the touch. There was discomfort, but not intense pain, for the first 12 hours, until they broke my water.

—Traci

I couldn't believe how much they hurt. I had been told all along that it was like a period cramp. But these were nothing like my period cramps. They were much sharper than a period cramp, but in the same spot.

—Sophia

They felt like someone was tying my stomach in knots.

—Maria

The contractions felt like menstrual cramps.

—Peggy

My contractions were whole belly—from top to bottom. Like some invisible hand was squeezing my belly.

—Grace

What surprised me was that I felt most of the pain in the front of my legs.

—Elizabeth

I wish I had known that I would be feeling pain in my buttocks, rather than my front.

—Lucy

My contractions were basically a painful tightening of my lower back that would radiate across my abdomen.

—Stephanie

I could feel the pain mostly in my hips—it was as though I was the wishbone on Thanksgiving and someone had each of my legs and was pulling them apart as hard as they could.

—Jasmine

TIP #9

....

DON'T BE SURPRISED IF CONTRACTIONS
START AND STOP, OR NEVER GET REGULAR

When I first went into labor, I knew it was different from the Braxton Hicks contractions I'd felt. These were either weak labor contractions or painful Braxton Hicks. However, they were 30 minutes apart, so I didn't worry. Over the next few days they became closer together and a little stronger, though not what I would consider painful. They stayed at 10 minutes apart for a few days. It was more annoying than anything else.

September 14, they became five minutes apart, lasting 45–60 seconds and they SEEMED to be painful. Two days later, they were STILL five minutes apart and I hadn't really progressed. My contractions had gotten uncomfortable and nearly as painful as the final ones—and they stayed that way. I stayed home and tried to wait for "real labor." The next day, my contractions more or less stopped.

I was looking forward to a good night's sleep when around 6:00 p.m. my contractions started up again painfully. Finally around 9:00 p.m., the contractions were about 6–7 minutes apart. When I got to the birth house, the midwife examined me. I was 8 cm dilated.

—Lisa

As the evening wore on, the pain of my contractions began to overtake me. As a defense against this pain, I slipped into a dreamlike state.

I fell into a deep slumber and awoke the next morning in a daze. It took me several moments to realize that my contractions had ceased. My labor must have stopped during the night.

—Katya

Lisa was 2 days overdue, so David and I decided to try some "natural" induction methods. At 8:30 p.m., about an hour later, I started to get mild contractions. I was a bit excited, but did not think anything was going on. They continued to come about 10 minutes apart for 2 hours or so. Even though I did not think it was "real" labor, we decided to pack our son's bag and send him to his grandparent's house for the night. Once I went to bed the contractions stopped completely.

—Heather

I felt very strange leaving the office, and I had a few contractions as I had earlier in the afternoon. I began timing them at 6:05, as they seemed to be getting closer together. I had another at 6:07 and they continued this way for the ENTIRE labor! This was very shocking to me, as I anticipated a delivery like I had learned about in childbirth class. You know—20 minutes apart for a few hours, 15 minutes and so on. I still thought I should go on a walk to get them on a more regular pattern. They would be 20 seconds long, then 30, back and forth.

—Suzanne

TIP #10

....

KEEP IN MIND THAT EARLY LABOR CAN LAST A LONG TIME—EVEN DAYS

I started having mild but regular contractions Sunday afternoon. I was so excited—finally I was in labor! As they were getting stronger and stayed regular, I went to the hospital. They said I was barely 1 cm dilated and sent me home. At home, the contractions were too painful to sleep so my husband and I walked around the neighborhood—all night long, practically. The next morning I went back to the hospital. I wasn't quite 2 cm dilated so they sent me home—again. At home, I bounced on the birthing ball, watched TV, walked more. That night I tried to sleep. Finally, Tuesday morning, the hospital finally admitted me. I was 3 cm dilated.

—Penny

I distinctly remember seeing the light begin to come up behind the shade in the room and thinking "What the heck is up with this? I have been in labor for TWO DAYS. I HAVE to get this baby out!"

—Shannon

I started cramping mildly on a Thursday evening. My doctor told me to come to the hospital when my contractions were 5 minutes apart, lasting for at least 60 seconds, for 1 hour. At about 10:00 p.m. I sat on the couch and timed my contractions. Most were about 5 minutes apart and lasted about 45-60 seconds. So, at 11:00 p.m., I woke my mom and told her it was time to go to the hospital. We got there around midnight and I was only 1 cm dilated, so my doctor told me to walk the halls all night and he'd come back in the morning.

I walked all night long. I knew every corner of the small rural hospital. My doctor came back around 7:00 a.m. I was still 1 cm, so he sent me home. I went home and slept off and on all day. My contractions spaced out and became irregular.

Around 10:00 p.m. my contractions were every 4–5 minutes and lasted about 60–90 seconds. They were definitely stronger than the night before. By the time we got back to the hospital my contractions were every 2–3 minutes and pretty intense. When my doctor finally got there, he said "You can stay. You're 5 cm."

—Casey

TIP #11

....

DON'T BE SURPRISED IF THE HOSPITAL WON'T READILY ADMIT YOU

On Tuesday night, I went to bed at about midnight feeling what I thought were the same type of contractions I had been having for weeks. At 2:30 a.m., I was woken up by the pain of a really bad contraction. It went away, so I tried to go back to sleep. Ten minutes later, I felt the same feeling again. By now I was starting to think, hey wait a minute, maybe I'm experiencing real contractions. I was starting to feel serious pain, but was so worried that I wasn't in labor at all. I didn't have any other symptoms, my water hadn't broke, I didn't experience any "bloody show," and the only other pain I had was a sharp pain in my vagina every 30 minutes or so. This went on until about 6:30 a.m., when I woke Devin up and told him we had better get to the hospital.

We got to the hospital only to discover that I had only dilated to 1 cm and my contractions were pretty far apart to be in active labor. They were still about 7 minutes apart, but the pain was excruciating. The nurse told me to walk for about an hour and see if that helped me progress. An hour later, I was 1.5 cm dilated. At about 11:00 a.m. they sent me home since I hadn't made any progress. They gave me a relaxant to help me sleep and told me to come back when the contractions got closer together.

—Jasmine

I felt some light contractions, about 10 minutes apart. I expected them to be Braxton Hicks. I have had them on and off over the last 2 weeks and had even been to the hospital once because they were 5 minutes apart.

After awhile I didn't notice the contractions anymore. That evening my husband and I were invited to a friend's house for dinner. About 1 hour before we had to go I felt the contractions again and timed them at about 7 minutes apart. So we went to my friend's house. The whole time there I had those contractions about every 7 minutes. I didn't want to go to the hospital again and be told it was a false alarm, so we decided to go for a walk and see if the contractions would stop or get stronger.

We walked for about 30 minutes and they kept coming. We decided to go see a movie ... my husband kept saying if we made some plans, then the baby was sure to come.

As we walked I felt the contractions coming on stronger. I told my husband I think I do want to go to the hospital. The doctor said I was 1 cm dilated and 80% effaced. Since they aren't allowed to admit me until I am 4 cm dilated, we had to go back home once again.

At 2 a.m. I got up because the pain was too bad to sleep. I tried watching TV. The contractions came about every 4–5 minutes and were VERY painful.

At 6:30 a.m. I was in so much pain I decided to wake up my husband. I told him "It hurts so bad, I want to go to the hospital." He said "OK," and fell back asleep.

I went into the shower and that's when I started bleeding. My husband finally got up and drove me back to the hospital. The doctor checked and I was finally 4 cm and 90% effaced, so they admitted me.

—Eve

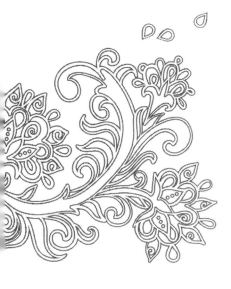

4 ADVICE AND ENCOURAGEMENT— WATER BREAKING

Some women think a big splash is going to usher in the big day—with lots of wet gushing drama and someone yelling "grab a towel, here she goes!"

Sorry to break it to you, girlfriend—but it's probably not going to happen that way. Many women are not sure the fluid leaking from them is amniotic fluid. If it is your water breaking, it could flow slowly or quickly. Or your doctor might have to break it in the hospital—like mine did, after my epidural.

Here is how water breaking often occurs:

- it could feel like a pop

- flow might be as light as a trickle

- or as heavy as a gush

- it often breaks before, during or after going to the bathroom

- it might not break on its own

TIP #12

....

YOUR WATER BREAKING MIGHT FEEL LIKE A "POP" BEFORE, DURING OR AFTER USING THE BATHROOM

The contractions weren't very strong, but after about 30 minutes down the highway, I had another contraction and I felt a "pop" around my upper abdomen. I thought perhaps my water had broken, but I didn't get the big gush of water.

When we arrived at the hospital, I mentioned that I thought my water broke and that I was possibly in labor. They made me pee in a cup and the results, according to them, were that it didn't break. So after hooking me up to the monitor, they called the doctor in to break it. When she got there, she gave me an exam and confirmed my belief that my water had broken. She said that the break was high and it didn't gush because the baby's head had stopped it from coming out.

—Rose

Around 8:45, I felt really nauseated and had to urinate (for about the 40th time that day), so I went to use the bathroom. As soon as I sat down, I knew something was different. I felt a discernible POP in my abdomen and suddenly fluid was rushing out of me—though I knew it wasn't urine! I called out to my husband, who was too engrossed in a TV program to hear me at first. I told him I was pretty sure my water had broken. That got his attention!

—Olivia

Around 4:00 p.m. my sister-in-law took me for a ride, to get me out of the house. We were going over some bumps on a dirt road and I said we better get home, I have to go to the bathroom. Truth was, I felt like I was going a little right there. As soon as I got out of the car I ran to the restroom. I was walking back to the couch and I felt like I had to go again, but this time fluid started coming out before I could make it to the bathroom. Sure enough, water was coming out sporadically ... not gushing but definitely a big leak.

I took a shower and we all headed to the hospital. When we got out of the car—that's when my water really broke. I was soaked.

—Lucy

Now my water broke at 5:00 p.m. while I was talking on the phone with my sister-in-law. I thought I had to go to the bathroom, so I got up, phone in hand, talking the whole time. Well it never stopped. I said I think my water broke because I thought I had to pee but I am still sitting here and it is still coming!

—Ayn

TIP #13

. . . .

YOUR WATER COULD STREAM OUT QUICKLY, LIKE A GUSH

I was 37 weeks along when on a Thursday morning at 4:30 I got up to use the restroom and when I thought I was finished, a big gush came out in the toilet. I did not know what that was. I just thought maybe I did not empty my bladder completely.

—Stella

Then I got up to go to the bathroom around 11:55. Tim had just turned off his light when I felt a gush—and I told him that my water just broke, and to please hurry and grab a towel. He jumped out of bed so fast! He was so excited! He got up and shaved, brushed his teeth, got our suitcases ready and called the insurance company. I called my doula, even though contractions had not yet begun. Tim also called his mom and dad. I got things ready for Rugger, our cat, and packed the last few things. We called the hospital and went in around 2:30 a.m. My water kept gushing!

—Allison

When we were about 3 minutes from the hospital, I felt a very weird "pop" inside me. My water had broken, but I didn't get the "gush" until I got out of the truck at the hospital.

—Cherise

TIP #14

....

OTHER WOMEN'S WATER EITHER TRICKLES OUT OR MUST BE "BROKEN" BY THE DOCTOR

I went to the grocery at 39 weeks. As I was going in I sneezed. I immediately felt wetness. I thought I had peed a little bit. When I returned home so I took a nap. My husband called, and I told him I peed in my pants; he had a good laugh and told his coworkers (so they could get a good laugh too). As I rolled over in bed, I felt more wetness. This was strange, and I wondered if the baby was pushing on my bladder. Not a lot of fluid, but enough to make you uncomfortable. This happened again 5 times in 5 minutes. I knew this could not be pee.

—Rosalind

Your water can break without a big gush. I was leaky with amniotic fluid for a week and a half before it was caught.

—Vicki

My water never broke on its own. After I had the epidural, my doctor had to "break" it. It was painless—I never felt a thing.

—Penny

I drank a ton of water at dinner, so I headed to the bathroom before dessert arrived. While in the potty, I felt a little more liquid come out than I expected. I looked in the toilet, and it was cloudy. I realized it could have been my water breaking, but it was just a leak. As we walked around the stores, I felt more leakage. When we got home, I went to the bathroom again and was positive it wasn't a random leak. I still wasn't having any contractions that I could feel.

—Lisa

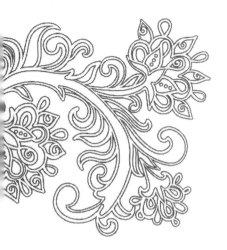

5   ADVICE AND ENCOURAGEMENT—
FAMILY AND FRIENDS

Family and friends can play a significant role in your labor and delivery. Unlike the old days when husbands and friends sat in the waiting room and waited and waited and waited, today the people close to you can help you give birth.

There are many ways husbands, family members, doulas or friends can comfort and assist you. They can:

- remind you of past victories

- brush your hair or let you squeeze an arm

- let you pull on a shirt

- remind you to sleep

TIP #15

············

FRIENDS AND FAMILY CAN REMIND YOU OF CHALLENGES YOU'VE OVERCOME

It was at this point that his encouragement became invaluable. He never let me give up. He kept reminding me that it was almost over, that I was doing so well. He reminded me of a challenging hiking trip we once took that needed a similar mental effort to complete. Even when all I wanted to do was give up and go to sleep he kept on being positive—exactly what I needed from him. He was the perfect birth partner for me.

—Meredith

TIP #16

. . . .

THEY CAN ALSO STROKE OR BRUSH YOUR HAIR AND REMIND YOU TO SLEEP

Once a contraction came on I felt myself drifting away from everything around me and was totally concentrated on my body. I developed an inner strength I didn't know I had and that's how I managed each one of the contractions. What really helped me was my husband stroking my hair or touching my hand while I had a contraction. I didn't want him to talk to me or to distract me. I just wanted to feel him close by.

—Eve

My husband was asleep in a fold out chair next to my bed and it kept getting later and later. I remember him and the nurses saying "Honey you better get some sleep so you have the energy to deliver this baby tomorrow."

—Marilyn

While I was sitting in the tub, my husband got my hairbrush and brushed my hair ... this was very relaxing and one of my favorite memories of the birth.

—Elizabeth

TIP #17

············

OR THEY CAN LET YOU PULL
ON THEIR SHIRT OR SQUEEZE AN ARM

*During the contractions the only thing that comforted me was pulling on
my husband's shirt.*

—Wendell

*When I was confined to a hospital bed, the only thing I wanted to do
during a contraction was squeeze my husband's forearm as hard as I could
and rock back and forth.*

—Andrea

*I tried the breathing exercises and they just made me dizzy and mad. It
did help to put my fingernails in my husband's arm when the pain got
too out of control.*

—Debbie

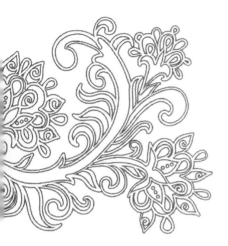

6 ADVICE AND ENCOURAGEMENT—
HANDLING LABOR PAIN

All women worry about the pain of labor. Even women bound for an epidural are anxious, since they are often not given until after women have been in labor for hours.

It doesn't help that pregnant women are often told different things. Books might instruct you to focus on your breathing, while your friend tells you to rock on a birthing ball.

You don't need a laundry list. You just need what works.

The main thing that helped me was a hot shower. Different methods, however, work for different women. The following is an assortment of pain-relief recommendations from new moms:

- · don't hold your breath

- · try a heated pad

- · ask that a nurse hold the fetal monitor on you *(with doctor's approval)*

- · have someone massage your back

- · walk around

- · take a bath or shower *(with doctor's approval)*

- · talk to the baby or rock in a rocking chair

- · try breathing exercises and focal points

TIP #18

....

BACK MASSAGES AND HEATED PADS CAN HELP EASE CONTRACTIONS

The thing that eased my labor pains most was having someone apply pressure to and massage my lower back. That helped an enormous amount. I don't know how I would have gotten through six hours of painful contractions without that.

—Stephanie

I'd had very bad back pain because my son was facing the wrong way. I used a rectangle-sized bean bag thingy, that you put in the microwave to heat. It really helped ease the constant back pain.

—Luciana

The thing that eased my labor pain the most was when I was squatting by the bed and the midwife pushed an area on my back in and down. It didn't eliminate the pain, but it made it SO much more bearable! Without her pushing on my back, the pain felt like it was just going all over the place. When she applied that pressure, it felt like the pain was going down and opening up my cervix like it was supposed to!

—Lisa

My nurse made me a hot pack for my back and that helped a lot.

—Sasha

TIP #19
. . . .

DON'T HOLD YOUR BREATH
DURING LABOR

I don't think there is anything I would have done differently, except listen to my mother more and breathe when she had told me to. I remember there were quite a few times where I would hold my breath, and that only made it worse.

—Isabella

As I was leaning onto hubby's shoulder for the epidural, my doctor entered the room. I remember her advising me to blow through one of the contractions. I did as instructed and found that the blowing really helped.

—Kristen

When a contraction started, I stared fixedly at the picture on the wall or focused on a window lever or some small speck or mark and just stared at it, looking at its detail and breathing through the sensations of pain and tightness. Breathing definitely helps. Holding your breath makes you tense and you feel the pain more. Forcing myself to keep puffing little shallow breaths in and out made a big difference.

—Lily

TIP #20

······

STAND OR WALK AROUND
AVOID LYING DOWN

(unless advised to stay still)

I couldn't deal with the pain while lying down. I was standing, walking, JUMPING up and down, or hopping from one foot to the other. It was silly, but for me, that was the only thing that helped.

—Vivian

I walked while I was in the early stages of labor and that helped ease the pain a little.

—Christine

I was most uncomfortable lying in bed. The only thing that really helped was to stand at the side of my bed rocking back and forth.

—Donna

TIP #21

. . . .

ASK TO HAVE A QUALIFIED PERSON HOLD THE FETAL MONITOR ON YOU SO YOU CAN MOVE AROUND

(unless advised to stay still)

Since I was 12 days late, the doctor was very cautious and put me on continuous fetal monitoring. The problem with this is that it usually requires that you stay in bed. However, because of a WONDERFUL nurse who served as our advocate, I was allowed some freedom to get up out of bed. She actually sat on the floor and held the monitor to my stomach while I labored in my husband's arm.

—Jane

They kept trying to put the fetal heart monitor elastic belts around my stomach, as they were concerned by the dipping heart rate. But my mind was starting to be in two places at once. On a conscious level, you felt you had to have the belt on to monitor your baby. On the other level, you were reduced to pure mammalian instinct and you wanted to shrug it off your skin, as it was constricting your stomach. In the end, the midwives took turns holding the end to my stomach to try to keep some form of contact with the heartbeat without using the belt.

—Lily

My doula was so helpful, though, she held all 3 monitors in place so I could labor in any position I wanted.

—Kim

TIP #22

. . . .

USING A ROCKING CHAIR
OR TALKING TO THE BABY CAN HELP

My contractions were manageable and I found that concentrating on breathing, walking, and rocking in a rocking chair all helped with pain management.

—Traci

In my second labor, I discovered that talking to the baby seemed to ease some of the pain. When a contraction came, I'd say out loud, "Good job baby! Come on out! I'm right here. We're in this together. I love you." Somehow, focusing on the baby rather than my pain helped a lot.

—Katya

Throughout early labor they had me try many different positions, but when the contractions were becoming more intense, I preferred to sit in a rocking chair with my feet in a pan of warm water.

—Allison

TIP #23

. . . .

BREATHING, MUSIC AND VISUALIZATION TECHNIQUES CAN HELP EASE CONTRACTIONS

We'd been listening to music pretty continuously since Sunday afternoon. My husband and I started with some simple breathing on Sunday evening when the contractions started to get painful. By midday on Monday, the focal point was out, and I needed help through the contractions. My husband guided my breathing when he could. I started sitting up in bed for every contraction and just rocking back and forth until it was over, then lying back in the bed. I think I even dozed in between the contractions, I was so worn out. My husband and I worked incredibly well together. He kept me focused away from the pain. The breathing really worked.

—Lisa

I used visualization techniques and I was able to relax through the pain. It didn't "go away" but I was able to make it through each one. I really was grateful for my labor music I had compiled throughout the last 8 months.

—Liz

The nurse reminded me of my breathing and it actually helped. It definitely didn't make the pain go away but it helped a little and gave me something to focus on other than the intense pain.

—Chyna

TIP #24

....

A BATH OR SHOWER CAN HELP THE PAIN
IF YOUR WATER HASN'T BROKEN

(not overly hot and with doctor's approval)

I walked all night but did not progress, although my contractions were so hard and unbearable. I asked for my epidural but the nurse said my contractions had to be closer and harder, even though I didn't think that was possible. She also told me to try the Jacuzzi, which was a lifesaver. It helped sooooo much and felt so good.

—Viola

I remember the only thing that helped was getting into the shower!

—Elizabeth

The hot water of the tub was heaven and really helped with the pain.

—Brianna

When I got to the hospital, the only thing that helped the pain of my contractions was a hot shower. I would first stand, and then when it really hurt I would sit on the seat in the shower and let the hot water run over me.

—Penny

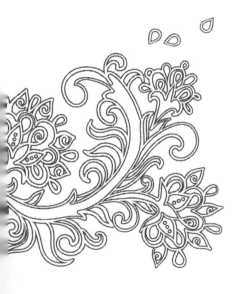

7 ADVICE AND ENCOURAGEMENT—
YOUR HOSPITAL STAY

Before I delivered, the only experiences I'd had with hospitals was visiting elderly relatives. So I had no idea what to expect. Would I be forced to share a bathroom? Could I have a private room or would nothing but a white curtain separate me from another woman's private moments?

Thankfully, while you cannot predict how your labor will unfold, you can and should make your hospital experience enjoyable. Think of it as an interior design-challenged hotel with attentive staff but bland food.

To prepare for your hospital stay, try to:

- visit the hospital beforehand

- limit the number of people in your room *(if commotion irritates you)*

- ask everyone to be quiet *(if noise bothers you)*

- let the nursery watch the baby so you can sleep *(if your hospital allows it)*

- have pillows in the car for the ride home

TIP #25

....

TOUR THE HOSPITAL'S
MATERNITY WARD BEFOREHAND

The hospital where I delivered encouraged pregnant women to tour the hospital as part of its pregnancy preparation class. I'm so happy I got to see the birthing rooms and nursery beforehand. When I was in the last trimester, I visualized myself giving birth in those rooms. I think that helped me feel not quite so nervous those last few weeks.

—Andrea

TIP #26

....

CONSIDER LIMITING
THE NUMBER OF PEOPLE IN YOUR ROOM

If I could do it differently I might not have told anyone that I was at the hospital (while I was in labor). All I wanted to do was take a nap, but I felt like everyone was there to see me, so I had to entertain.

—Deanna

If I had to do it all over again, I would limit the visitors in my room. I had originally said my mother, stepmother, mother-in-law and (of course) husband could be in the room during birth. However, now that I know the pain and how annoying people can be, I would not allow anyone except my husband, mother and stepmother. Next time around, I will make it clear to the staff that these are the only people allowed unless I ask for someone else.

—Cathy

TIP #27

. . . .

LET THE NURSERY WATCH
THE BABY AT NIGHT SO YOU CAN SLEEP
(if your hospital allows it)

When my son cried all night after he was born, I should have pushed the call button and DEMAND that they take him for a few hours while I got some rest, as I was about to lose it. I can't believe I did not want to bother them. Ay ay ay!

—Stella

My sister gave me some great advice. She said to take advantage of the nursery the hospital provides, especially at night. When I wanted my daughter with me, all I did was call and have her brought in. But when I needed to get some sleep, I had them take her out (although I tried to sneak a peek into the nursery at night to make sure she was OK). They brought her in to breastfeed a few times in the night. But it was great getting a little rest in between.

—Penny

TIP #28

. . . .

SHUSH—A QUIET ROOM
HAS HELPED SOME WOMEN

During this entire time everything and everyone had been quiet and serene—I would quicken my breathing-out during the contractions and then slow it down in between—no moaning, no sounding—just peace and quiet. At one point I heard my nephew start to cry and immediately asked for him to leave—but he was already out the door by that point. I remember one nurse was so excited that she wanted to be "encouraging" during my contractions—everyone told her to keep quiet and I was able to zone her out.

—Heather

I remember at one point telling everyone I didn't want to do this anymore and I was going home. I was mean to my nurses and family. Cursing at them to be quiet. When in severe pain, I learned, I needed quiet. My poor mother's hand became all bruised and my sister must have smoked 3 packs of cigarettes. My father was at a local bar calling the room every 5 minutes wanting updates.

During extreme contractions I would hold on tight to the bed and close my eyes and breathe. It HAD to be quiet.

—Yolanda

In my first labor, complete silence also helped because it allowed me to slip into that amazing birthing reverie where pain is less sharp and noticeable.

—Katya

TIP #29

············

THROW SOME PILLOWS IN THE CAR
FOR THE RIDE HOME

I wish someone would have told my husband to bring pillows to sit on for the ride home. I can't stress that enough. I was warned pretty much about everything else, but no one told me how painful riding in the car would be.

—Andrea

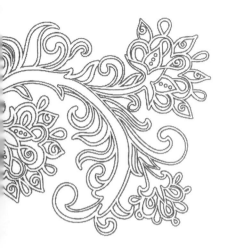

8   ADVICE AND ENCOURAGEMENT—
EPIDURALS

As the pregnancy progresses and the baby gets bigger and BIGGER and **BIGGER**—even the most laid-back woman will wonder how she's going to get the baby out. Talk about a square peg through a round hole—that's nothing compared to this. Little opening + big head equals *oy vey*.

The answer for many women is an epidural. But how hard is it to get the needle in? Must it really be stuck in your spine, of all places? Does it always work?

Relax—epidurals are safe and effective for most women. Here are some women's experiences:

· epidurals usually work great

· they sometimes either speed up or slow down dilation

· don't move while they put it in

· you will still be expected to push

· don't get one if you want to be up and around quickly

TIP #30

············

RELAX—
EPIDURALS USUALLY WORK

By about 2:45 a.m., the nurse said if I wanted an epidural, she could call the doctor. She said she had never seen someone have so many contractions this close together before. I received the epidural, and that was the best thing ever invented. I couldn't stop telling the nurse how much I loved her.

—Beth

After about an hour of hard contractions, I finally got my epidural and it was smooth sailing from there. My epidural took effect and was great! I took a couple of naps, talked on the phone, watched TV. It was great— family had time to come and visit and go to the waiting room. The nurse came in at about 9:45 p.m. and checked my dilation, and said I was fully dilated and effaced.

—Olivia

I got the epidural as soon as possible and it was GREAT! I thought I was going to be nervous when he put the needle in my spine, but I was so ready for the pain relief that I was not nervous at all! I began to be at ease, thinking this is OK. It won't be so bad. I was joking and laughing with family and friends.

—Brooke

TIP #31

....

EPIDURALS SOMETIMES SPEED UP
OR SLOW DOWN DILATION

After the epidural, I felt contractions but not pain. This was the best I'd felt in over 24 hours. But within an hour the epidural was wearing off of my left side. The anesthesiologist gave me another dose.

The second dose knocked out all sensation. I couldn't move my legs or feet. The nurse announced that I had dilated to 7 cm. I was surprised at how quickly I'd gone from 4 to 7 cm, since I'd read that epidurals tend to slow down labor, not accelerate it.

—Kristen

My doctor said I could get my epidural. Thank goodness! Around 3:15 a.m. the doctor came in and did my epidural, and boy did I feel better. They kept telling us I would probably have the baby in a few hours, but then the contractions started to slow down. And it kept getting later so we told everyone to go home and sleep and come back in the morning. Finally I fell asleep and my poor husband made himself a place on the floor and tried to sleep too.

—Rose

The nurse checked me and I was at 5 cm. The epidural guy came. I had strong contractions while he was administering the epidural, but I said to myself this is the last contraction I'm going to feel, so just stay still. The epidural started working almost immediately. I didn't feel anything. Within 10 minutes of getting the epidural the nurse checked and I was at 8 cm! The epidural got me to relax, so I progressed quickly.

—Jessica

TIP #32

. . . .

HOLD STILL AND CURL UP
WHILE THEY PUT THE NEEDLE IN

After it seemed like FOREVER for the anesthesiologist to get there, he finally arrived. I was so excited. The pain would be over. When he was trying to give me the epidural, it seemed like he was taking forever. Finally, after a few minutes, he announced he didn't think he could get it in. What! What was the problem? He said it might help if I curled up really tight (I guess to make my spine stand out). I was in so much pain, but in desperation I curled up so well, he got it in almost immediately. I wish he'd told me that at the beginning!

—Penny

When the doctor finally came in to give me my epidural, I was so scared I would flinch during a contraction. The pain was too much to sit perfectly still. A large nurse promised me she would not let me move. She then ordered everyone out of the room. She laid on top of me as the epidural was administered. Just as she promised, I didn't move! I don't think I could have moved if my life depended on it.

—Maria

TIP #33

....

BELIEVE IT OR NOT
YOU CAN PUSH EVEN WHEN NUMB

*Later, when I was fully dilated, the epidural was switched off, to allow
me to regain some feeling for the pushing. Unfortunately (or perhaps for-
tunately), the dose had been so high that I was completely numb from ribs
to toes. I couldn't even move my legs. Since I couldn't feel anything at all,
I put my hand on my belly and watched the monitor in order to know
when a contraction was starting. When the contraction began I drew a
deep breath, pushed the extra air down into my lungs, and pushed. I
couldn't feel the place where I was pushing, but imagined my perineum
and concentrated on that area.*

—Kristen

*I was so numb from the epidural, I was surprised that my doctor asked
me to push. Push? I can't feel anything. He told me to imagine where my
cervix was and concentrate on bearing down hard in that spot when he
told me. It was so strange because I couldn't feel much. I tried to imagine
what my body should be doing and tried to make it do that even though
I couldn't feel my muscles push. But apparently it worked because I only
had to push about 40 minutes.*

—Andrea

TIP #34

....

IF YOU WANT TO BE UP AND AROUND SOON CONSIDER NOT HAVING AN EPIDURAL

After going through labor without an epidural, I would have done the first one that way too. I felt so much better after. I was up and playing with Nicholas outside two days after I had Jacob.

—Grace

Knowing all I do about what an unmedicated birth feels like—I'll definitely have another natural labor next time. The biggest advantage was I felt well enough to go home four hours after giving birth.

—Lisa

9 ADVICE AND ENCOURAGEMENT— WOMEN NOT GETTING AN EPIDURAL

Many women plan to birth their babies naturally, without an epidural. Women delivering pain medication-free should prepare early. As soon as possible, make a plan for handling the pain, assemble a team of family members and/or a facilitator (such as a midwife or doula) and arm yourself with coping techniques.

The pain-relief options discussed in chapter 6 will help with an epidural-free delivery. Here is additional advice from women who chose natural childbirth:

- practice relaxation techniques beforehand

- prepare hospital staff by giving them a "no epidural" birth plan

- consider a water birth *(controversial and not available in many hospitals or facilities)*

- it might help to talk and chant

- focus on your task and don't be afraid—your body is meant to do this

TIP #35

....

MAKE SURE YOU PRACTICE
RELAXATION TECHNIQUES BEFOREHAND

The fact that I had been practicing relaxation and listening to my hypno-birth [lessons] every day made it a lot easier to stay relaxed during transition. I wouldn't have been able to do it without pain medication if I had not been practicing.

—Peggy

TIP #36

. . . .

GIVE HOSPITAL STAFF YOUR
"NO EPIDURAL" BIRTH PLAN IMMEDIATELY

We made it clear not to offer me an epidural, and the nurses never suggested anything of the sort.

—Amy

I said in my birth plan that I didn't want them to offer me drugs, and I'm so glad they didn't.

—Lisa

TIP #37

....

CONSIDER A WATER BIRTH

(controversial and not available in many hospitals or facilities)

I had been sitting in the bath to ease my contractions (FABULOUS) and decided I wasn't getting out. So my midwife (bless her) organized another nurse to come in and we had a water birth instead. This was totally unplanned but exactly what I needed at the time. The water delivery was no less painful, but the water allowed me to move around more easily and I felt more comfortable during the contractions.

—Margi

I don't think there is any information I wished I had had beforehand, although I wish I had heard of a water birth for my first one.

—Elizabeth

TIP #38

....

TALKING OUT LOUD
CAN HELP THE PAIN

As the contractions intensified, I used my voice more. I chanted "I'm opening" or "open up" to connect with what my cervix was doing and needed to do more of. I continued with "Ohhh" sounds as well, dragging the sound out to the peak of the contraction.

Lauren and Kim parked while I headed for the emergency room. As soon as I stepped through the doors, I felt another contraction coming. This was the ONLY time during my labor that I didn't "let my monkey [codeword for vocalizing] do it." I was standing in front of a coffee kiosk with a line of folks, so I leaned against a wall and just did my breathing. I didn't want to vocalize in front of those people, as it probably would have freaked them out. After it was over, I opened my eyes and the coffee guy said kindly, "Are you all right, ma'am?" I said I was, and toddled off to admitting.

—Amy

When a contraction came on, I'd say out loud, "Good job baby! Come on out! I'm right here. We're in this together. I love you." Somehow, focusing on the baby rather than my pain helped a lot.

—Katya

I was continually walking around the house, stopping to "dance" during my contractions. I would chant "baby's coming, baby's coming" during each contraction, which helped far more than the breathing I had learned.

—Cherise

TIP #39

···········

DON'T BE AFRAID—YOUR BODY IS MADE TO GIVE BIRTH WITHOUT DRUGS

A big part of it is mental. It's all a mind game to tell yourself it's not the end of the world. The contraction will end and there are a few minutes of respite before the next one. I just kept telling myself the whole thing will end. Remaining concentrated and focused is important. Not being afraid of it is also very important. Contractions hurt, but they can't kill you and they will end.

—Meredith

I would like to be able to give every first-time pregnant mom these bits of info: You Can Do It. Your body was made for it, it will do what needs to be done if you relax and stay out of the way. Don't be afraid...fear equals pain. It is only a few hours, or a day (or 2 or 3), out of the many days of your life.

—Elizabeth

The other thing I knew before my first labor that helped me immensely is something my mother told me (she was a childbirth instructor for many years)—that women in comas are allowed to birth vaginally. Their bodies know what to do, and because they are unaware of pain (hopefully), their minds do not get in the way to complicate things. Their bodies take over and they birth their babies. I figured—if they can do it—so can I!

—Katya

I just kept reminding myself what our childbirth instructor kept saying—it's only one day of your life. Anyone can withstand pain for one day. It was more like two for me, but I still knew there was an end to the madness.

—Lisa

Your body was meant to do this. Your body won't ask more of you than you can handle.

—Jane

10 ADVICE AND ENCOURAGEMENT— C-SECTIONS

The rate of women having children via Caesarean section is at a record high. And because some of these C-sections weren't planned but occurred due to unforeseen complications in a vaginal delivery, all women should prepare for the possibility of a C-section.

I want your birthing experience to go smoothly. **Every woman, therefore, should read this section.**

Here are things you can do to make a C-section more comfortable:

- don't worry—it goes smoothly for most women

- bring a small blanket and music

- expect to feel pressure, tugging or nothing at all

- ask beforehand that your baby be brought to you quickly

- move around as soon as your doctor will allow

- consider using silicone strips, which could reduce scarring

TIP #40

. . . .

DON'T WORRY—THE C-SECTION SURGERY AND RECOVERY GO SMOOTHLY FOR MOST WOMEN

My recovery after my C-section was not that bad. I have heard a lot of bad things about how much it hurts, but I was off the morphine pump and able to move around easily the next day. My staples were taken out a week after the surgery. The doctor who delivered my son used a laser to make the incision. It healed and now looks barely visible.

—Heidi

Oh! And the C-section was not as bad as everything I read said. It hurt, but I expected way worse.

—Lucia

The doctors and nurses were wonderful. My long-feared C-section went very smoothly.

—Marilyn

TIP #41

....

CONSIDER BRINGING A SMALL BLANKET TO THE HOSPITAL

Soon after the surgery, I began having major chills, couldn't get warm enough. I'm told that's a common side effect from the spinal.

—Chantal

I remember my face itching and being very cold, which they said were side effects from the spinal and were normal.

—Marilyn

TIP #42

. . . .

MUSIC COULD HELP
EASE LAG TIME

I wish someone suggested I bring along music. Everything seemed to take such a long time, and I got bored just lying there. It would have been great to listen to my favorite band.

—Delia

TIP #43

. . . .

YOU MIGHT FEEL PRESSURE OR TUGGING
OR ALMOST NOTHING

Once surgery started things happened very quickly. The doctor said it would feel like an elephant pressing on my chest when they pulled the baby out, so I had prepared myself for that. I ended up feeling very little pressure. I wasn't even aware my son had been born until he started crying.

—Stephanie

I only felt pressure and then got to see my beautiful son.

—Marilyn

The C-section was not a bad experience for me at all. I did not feel a thing during the surgery, but a lot of pressure. And some tugging and pulling. I can't quite explain it. There is no pain, but a lot of tugging. The whole thing lasted less than half an hour.

—Julia

TIP #44

. . . .

ASK TO HAVE THE BABY BROUGHT TO YOU
AS SOON AS POSSIBLE AFTER THE C-SECTION

I should have done more research about what would happen right after the C-section. I was disappointed that I didn't get to see my son for so long after the surgery. I know many hospitals let the babies stay with the mom while the doctors are finishing the surgery. I think I should have tried to have a plan in place ahead of time.

—Stephanie

TIP #45

. . . .

TRY TO GET MOVING AS QUICKLY AS
YOUR DOCTOR WILL ALLOW AFTERWARDS

The recovery from a C-section was not physically that painful, but it was intense. I had a speedy recovery, but it is very important to take the pain meds so that you can move about. And I took some stuff for gas. It is true that you need to be up and about as soon as you can after surgery.

—Carolyn

The next morning I was told I should try sitting on the edge of the bed and dangling my legs. That wasn't hard at all so I decided to get up and walk. That was a little harder. I decided to hold a pillow against the incision as it felt like my insides would fall out if I didn't. I walked stooped over for the first day or so. I tried to stay out of bed as much as possible as they said that would speed my recovery.

—Stephanie

I plan to have a repeat C-section with my next child and I definitely now know what to expect and what to do to speed up my recovery—get up and move around as soon as you can!

—Chantal

TIP #46

············

GOOD NEWS—SILICONE STRIPS COULD LESSEN SCARRING

I'm so glad my doctor recommended a silicone strip to help the incision heal better and scar less. I just bought the cheap ones from the drugstore and I barely have any visible scar now.

—Mia

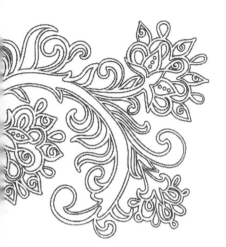

11 ADVICE AND ENCOURAGEMENT—
BREASTFEEDING

Women who choose breast over bottle feeding should know that although breastfeeding is a natural way to feed an infant, the process doesn't always come naturally. Also, situations can arise that could make nursing difficult. The good news is that techniques for effective breastfeeding are not difficult to learn.

Although not a complete guide to breastfeeding, here are some women's nursing advice:

· bring nursing pillow to hospital

· use lanolin cream

· try to breastfeed almost immediately

· learn "quick latch" technique

· gently pull out baby's lips *(if they curl in)*

· breastfeed consistently

TIP #47

. . . .

BRING YOUR NURSING PILLOW
TO THE HOSPITAL

I wish I would have brought my nursing pillow to the hospital so I could get used to nursing with it.

—Bertha

TIP #48

. . . .

SLATHER LANOLIN CREAM
ON NIPPLES AFTER NURSING

I'm so glad the hospital had given me lanolin cream. I was able to prevent my nipples from chafing or getting too sore by putting it on each nipple and areola immediately after Brooke nursed (and even after she switched nipples). This chance bit of advice about lanolin cream is what helped me most the first few weeks.

—Andrea

TIP #49

. . . .

NURSE SOON
AND CONSISTENTLY AFTER DELIVERY

One thing I greatly regret. I wish I would have demanded to breastfeed her right after her birth. The doctor said that placing the baby on my tummy was just ceremonial. I didn't even get a chance to look at or inspect her. My baby ended up not breastfeeding well and dropped more than 10% of her body weight. They made me supplement. I wish I would have known this could happen, and how important the immediate afterbirth time was.

—Darwati

What would I have done differently? Although I tried breastfeeding, I wasn't really consistent so I ended up with severe engorgement. I wish I had been more consistent in how I fed the baby in the hospital.

—Jeannette

I had a hard time breastfeeding my daughter because I didn't nurse her for a long time after delivery. Soon after I had her, she slept for the longest time. In the interim, my milk came in. Since I didn't want to wake her up, my breasts became so engorged that when I finally tried to nurse her she couldn't latch on because they were so hard. I wish I would have nursed her sooner (even waking her up to do it) or pumped after my milk came in.

—Penny

TIP #50

. . . .

THE SECRET TO
A GOOD LATCH IS ...

One of the secrets to a good "latch" is to quickly place your baby's wide open mouth onto your breast in one fast motion, so you get all or most of your areola in. Also, after he was latched on, I pressed down slightly on my breast just above his nose, so I was sure he could breathe (for the first week or so, when his face was tiny). I also pulled out his lips so they weren't tucked inside his mouth.

—Andrea

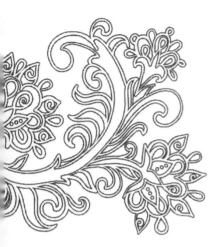

FUN
REAL-LIFE STORIES

Yes, there can be humor in childbirth.

Sit. Enjoy a laugh or two. You deserve it.

Chick-fil-A server exclaimed "Is she going to have that baby here?!"

> *My mom and I walked that afternoon (we were enjoying the great May weather). I started having regular contractions around 6:00 p.m. My husband and I decided to go to the mall to see if the contractions were "real." He needed new tennis shoes. At the beginning of the trip I wasn't in much pain, but towards the end of the trip I was in a lot of pain. Bruce, my husband, wanted to get some dinner so we stopped at a Chick-fil-A. I didn't want anything (which is weird because Chick-fil-A is my favorite!) and while he was ordering (at this time it was around 8:45) I had a major contraction. I leaned against the counter so I could breathe and the girl behind the counter said "Is she going to have that baby here?!" and I wanted to say "YES—I love Chick-fil-A SO much I want to have my first born in one!"*

> —Grace

"Sorry I'm so hairy!"

> *As I was crowning, and Baby A (William) was right there, the nurse told me to feel his head. I did and it was really strange. I was then moved to an operating room to continue to deliver. It was crazy—I had to move from the birthing bed to the operating table with a head between my legs. As I was pushing William out, I noticed there were about 30 people in the operating room. I asked why and was told*

that I had five doctors and nurses, each baby had five doctors and nurses and the rest were students (it was a teaching hospital) needing credit to see a vaginal twin delivery. I was so happy (NOT) to be a class project. All I could think of was, I had not shaved in five months and I kept apologizing to everyone in the room for how hairy I was.

—Jennifer

She sent her friends out for "good" toilet paper and her favorite restaurant snack.

I walked into the bathroom at the hospital to change and realized I had forgotten my Charmin, so without another word the doula was off to the store for the "good" toilet paper—a must in my book! Later on, once we got back to my room I had the nurse start filling up the tub. I was also getting hungry by then so I sent my brother to Outback Steakhouse to get me a loaded baked potato.

—Heather

You want me to weigh *what?*

We decided that maybe my water had broken so we called and they said to go to the hospital. Again I was confused, I thought that when your water broke you could go sailing, not just feel like you peed on yourself—but hey who was I to know. We showed up at the hospital and she wanted to know exactly how many pads I had soaked and what they weighed. At this moment I saw the science in it and pictured myself in my kitchen weighing my maxi pad on the gram scale I didn't own. Clueless, I told her I had not counted my pads and I didn't weigh them, that's for sure. The nurse looked at me as if all pregnant women were supposed to know to weigh their pads!

—Vicki

Nurse lifts sheet to find head sticking out—surprise!

I woke up around 11:00 a.m. and asked for an epidural. They checked me at 9 cm and immediately called for my doctor to come. She did not make it in time. I told the nurse I could feel the head (I meant that I could feel the head coming out of me). The nurse lifted up the sheet and his head was all the way out. A few seconds later his shoulders were out. I did not push once.

My husband was the first to know that it was a boy. He was so excited. The doctor came running in a minute later. A few minutes after giving birth I was sitting up, eating some fruit and cheese, and happily nursing my son.

I was in labor for 3 hours and 51 minutes from the start of Pitocin, 2 hours and 41 minutes from the start of contractions. I had no tears. He was born while we listened to "Only Women Bleed" by Alice Cooper.

—Amber

"What do you want on your pizza, doctor?"

I had been pushing every 30-60 seconds for an hour. I felt like I had run a marathon, but no progress seemed to have been made. My husband would occasionally give me an ice chip to suck on—the only liquid I could have. The nurse told my husband to look down so he could see the baby's head—apparently she was quite hairy. I wanted no part of this. I could feel what was happening, and that was gruesome enough.

At some point, someone popped their head in the door and asked what my nurse and doctor wanted on their pizza.

—Brenda

"Hold that baby in until I get this glove on!"

Mom told the doctor that she thought things were progressing fast and she thought the doctor should stay for a little bit. The doctor didn't believe my mom and told her that I was only dilated to a 6 and it would be a while. During their conversation, I just couldn't believe that I was only dilated to a 6. I reached down to check myself and I felt Lisa's head! I kind of yelped and the doctor and my mom came back in. All I could say is "the baby is coming!" The doctor turned on the light and said she would check me herself. She looked down in the bathtub and yelled "Oh my gosh! Is that a head? Hurry! We're having a baby now!" All of a sudden everyone was running around like crazy! They started to pull the delivery cart over to the bathroom to deliver the baby in the tub, but then the contraction stopped. With the help of my mom and a nurse, I got out of the bathtub and kind of "flew" to the bed. As I sat down on the bed, Lisa's head was born. Everyone was yelling for help and the doctor yelled at the nurse "hold that baby in until I get this glove on!" Just as the doctor pulled the second glove on, Lisa was born and the doctor literally "caught her."

—Liz

Interesting movie choice during labor

We had on the "Thomas Crown Affair" during one part of our stay. Just like when you were little and your father walks into the makeout scene of a movie, the anesthesiologist was putting in the needle just as the two main characters starting dirty dancing and then having sex. Awkward moment. My husband and I both joked that we should have said, "No, we are not watching porn." Next time I'm bringing "Finding Nemo."

—Chyna

EPILOGUE

Finally, some parting words for you, dear friend, who is about to experience the most incredible event of your life. In the end, it's all worth it. Your life will never be the same. Enjoy these sweet reflections about the wondrous and miraculous joy of bringing new life into the world:

The love I have for my daughter could never, ever, ever be explained in words. She is my life. She is the coolest thing that has ever happened to me. I cannot ever imagine being without her.

—Shannon

I think the feeling of having a child is so unbelievably joyous. If you could bottle it up, it would be the best selling drug ever.

—Wendi

It was a magnificent feeling to hold that little boy in my arms.

—Charlotte

Seeing my baby girl for the first time and witnessing the miracle of her life was the greatest thing I have ever known and I am reminded of it every day when I look into her eyes and she smiles right back at me.

—Isabella

I can't imagine life without him now. Sometimes, while I'm watching him play or sleep or run around the house being his silly self, I have to stop for just a minute because he literally takes my breath away. I've told my husband that before, but he just looks at me. I think it's a feeling only a mommy can understand.

—Angelika

The world was perfect at that moment—the three of us now a seamless, impenetrable family. I was happy and whole and deeply in love with my daughter and husband and eternally grateful to the women who were present to witness this amazing event. At that moment, the ground beneath us shook momentarily—an earthquake celebrating our daughter's arrival. And I understood for the first time the power of my being, the depth of my connection to this Earth and the wonder of this existence.

—Katya

The best part of this story is that it's two years later and I am ready to do it all again! It's amazing how these little ones change your life and attitude towards things. Only a blessing from above!

—Carol

ACKNOWLEDGEMENTS

I would like to thank a number of people. First and foremost, to the moms who took time out of their busy lives to send me their birth stories—my most heartfelt thank you! Because of you, countless women will have information, advice and encouragement we did not have. I pray this book will encourage and embrace expectant mothers everywhere, some of whom may be giving birth without their moms, sisters, grandmothers or significant others.

May these pregnant women think of us as their surrogate family during this time—because we are. Hopefully they will feel us holding their hands—because we will be.

Second, I would like to thank my children. If I hadn't been in early labor nearly 2 days with my first born, this book would never have been written. Allison—thanks for tenaciously holding on. Maybe theater mommy was showing cheerleading routines, over and over. I hope you two spend your entire lives close by, holding on. And gainfully employed.

Thank you babycenter.com—for enabling me to reach the women who responded to my request for birth stories.

Thank you Traci. Whenever I felt overwhelmed by the difficulty of this enormous project, I could always count on you for encourage-ment and friendship. If you'd been around since the beginning, it might not have taken 10 years. And I'm sorry I had to change the cover. You will forever be featured inside and on the back cover — belly, baby and all!

Thanks also to my family, husband and friends. Vance, Carol and Lis—for your support and advice. Elizabeth, Dar, Jeannette and Greg—you are my rocks, my patient and faithful sounding boards and my extended family.

I also want to thank my team of designers for making this dream a reality. Thank you Josh, Susanne, Teri, Lynne and Bridget for sticking with it and not disconnecting your phones and computers. You are artists with unending patience and good hearts.

Lastly, I need to thank the literary agents who rejected my book. You gave me the courage to go back to the drawing board, make the book better and ultimately do it myself. I think it's a better book because of it.

LIST OF TIPS

TIP #1   Bring magazines, a camera and a small mirror to the hospital

TIP #2   Don't forget nice clothes for everyone, your favorite soap and baggy pants

TIP #3   Pack a maternity nightgown and your favorite socks

TIP #4   You'll also need breast pads, lip balm and your nursing bra *(if you're breastfeeding)*

TIP #5   Stimulating nipples can bring on labor *(with doctor's approval)*

TIP #6   Intercourse or walking can stimulate contractions

TIP #7   Some women use breast pumps to induce labor *(with doctor's approval)*

TIP #8   Realize that contractions feel different to different people

TIP #9   Don't be surprised if contractions start and stop, or never get regular

TIP #10 Keep in mind that early labor can last a long time— even days

TIP #11 Don't be surprised if the hospital won't readily admit you

TIP #12 Your water breaking might seem like a "pop" before, during or after using the bathroom

TIP #13   Your water could stream out quickly, like a gush

TIP #14   Other women's water either trickles out or must be "broken"
          by the doctor

TIP #15   Friends and family can remind you of challenges you've
          overcome

TIP #16   They can also stroke or brush your hair and remind you
          to sleep

TIP #17   Or they can let you pull on their shirt or squeeze an arm

TIP #18   Back massages and heated pads can help ease contractions

TIP #19   Don't hold your breath during labor

TIP #20   Stand or walk around—avoid lying down *(unless advised
          to stay still)*

TIP #21   Ask to have a qualified person hold the fetal monitor on
          you so you can move around *(unless advised to stay still)*

TIP #22   Using a rocking chair or talking to the baby can help

TIP #23   Breathing, music and visualization techniques can help ease
          contractions

TIP #24 A bath or shower can help the pain if your water hasn't broken *(not overly hot and with doctor's approval)*

TIP #25 Tour the hospital's maternity ward beforehand

TIP #26 Consider limiting the number of people in your room

TIP #27 Let the nursery watch the baby at night so you can sleep *(if your hospital allows it)*

TIP #28 Shush—a quiet room has helped some women

TIP #29 Throw some pillows in the car for the ride home

TIP #30 Relax—epidurals usually work

TIP #31 Epidurals sometimes speed up or slow down dilation

TIP #32 Hold still and curl up while they put the needle in

TIP #33 Believe it or not, you can push even when numb

TIP #34 If you want to be up and around soon, consider not having an epidural

TIP #35 Make sure you practice relaxation techniques beforehand

TIP #36 Give hospital staff your "no epidural" birth plan immediately

TIP #37 Consider a water birth *(controversial and not available in many hospitals or facilities)*

TIP #38 Talking out loud can help the pain

TIP #39 Don't be afraid—your body is made to give birth without drugs

TIP #40 Don't worry—the C-section surgery and recovery go smoothly for most women

TIP #41 Consider bringing a small blanket to the hospital

TIP #42 Music could help ease lag time

TIP #43 You might feel pressure or tugging—or almost nothing

TIP #44 Ask to have the baby brought to you as soon as possible after the C-section

TIP #45 Try to get moving as quickly as your doctor will allow afterwards

TIP #46 Good news—silicone strips could lessen scarring

TIP #47 Bring your nursing pillow to the hospital

TIP #48 Slather lanolin cream on nipples after nursing

TIP #49 Nurse soon and consistently after delivery

TIP #50 The secret to a good latch is ...

♡

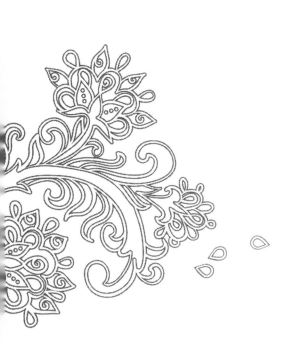

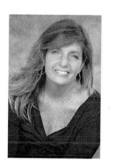

AUTHOR

Pamela Peery is a former lawyer, legal editor and law professor. She lives in Southern California with her family and loves rock climbing when she can steal away for a few minutes.

NOTES

NOTES

NOTES